NEAPOLITAN MASTIFF DOG

The Complete Handbook On How To Raising And Caring For Neapolitan Mastiff Dog

I0427465

CHAD BRUNO

Table of Contents

Introductory

The Neapolitan Mastiff, also known as the Mastino Napoletano, is a huge and historic breed of dog that originated in Italy. These dogs are recognized for their intimidating and unusual appearance. Here are some significant qualities and information about the Neapolitan Mastiff:

1. Appearance: Neapolitan Mastiffs are big, muscular dogs with loose, wrinkled skin. They have a deep, broad head with a flat skull and a unique, deeply wrinkled face. Their eyes are small and firmly set, and their ears are trapezoidal and hang down. The breed has a short, dense coat that comes in numerous hues, including gray, blue, black, tawny, and mahogany.

2. Size: These dogs are huge and heavy. Adult Neapolitan Mastiffs normally weigh between 140 to 150 pounds (63 to 68 kilograms) or more, and they stand from 24 to 31 inches (61 to 79 centimeters) at the shoulder.

3. Temperament: Neapolitan Mastiffs are recognized for their protective and devoted attitude. They are typically described as gentle giants and are highly dedicated to their families. They can be reticent and aloof with strangers, which makes them great guard dogs. Proper socialization and training are vital to guarantee they are well-behaved and don't become unduly aggressive.

4. History: The Neapolitan Mastiff has a long history, stretching back to ancient Roman times. They were initially bred for numerous functions, including defending property and cattle. Their striking appearance and protective instincts have made them a sought-after breed for decades.

5. Care & Maintenance: Due to their size and wrinkled skin, Neapolitan Mastiffs require specific care. Regular cleaning and care of their skin folds are required to prevent skin infections. These dogs also need plenty of exercise and mental stimulation to keep them happy and healthy. Because of their size, they may not be ideal for tiny living spaces.

6. Health: Like many huge breeds, Neapolitan Mastiffs might be prone to various health conditions, including hip dysplasia, bloat, and skin problems due to their wrinkles. Responsible breeding and frequent veterinarian care can help alleviate some of these difficulties.

7. Lifespan: Neapolitan Mastiffs normally have a lifespan of roughly 7 to 9 years.

It's crucial to investigate and understand the demands and features of Neapolitan Mastiffs completely before selecting them as a companion. They require proper training, socialization, and care to be well-adjusted and healthy companions.

CHAPTER ONE
Neapolitan Mastiff Characteristics

Neapolitan Mastiffs have various specific qualities that set them different from other dog breeds. Here are some of the important traits of Neapolitan Mastiffs:

1. Large and Muscular Build: Neapolitan Mastiffs are recognized for their enormous and muscular bodies. They are a very hefty breed with a muscular and imposing presence.

2. Distinctive Wrinkled Skin: The most remarkable trait of Neapolitan Mastiffs is their loose, wrinkled skin. These deep wrinkles and folds, especially on their forehead and neck, give them a unique and terrifying aspect.

3. Powerful Head: They have a wide, broad head with a flat skull. Their face is extremely wrinkled, with loose skin producing folds around the eyes and muzzle.

4. Short Coat: Neapolitan Mastiffs have a short, dense coat that is normally smooth and can come in numerous hues, including gray, blue, black, tawny, and mahogany.

5. Droopy Ears: Their ears are trapezoidal in shape and dangle down close to their cheeks.

6. Scary Appearance: Their entire appearance, with the combination of their size, wrinkled skin, and unusual head shape, makes them look scary and serves as a deterrent to potential intruders.

7. Protective and Loyal: Neapolitan Mastiffs are recognized for their devotion and protective temperament. They are frequently dedicated to their families and can be great security dogs, as they are instinctively distrustful of strangers.

8. Reserved with Strangers: While they are loyal to their owners, Neapolitan Mastiffs can be reserved and aloof with strangers, which is a feature that contributes to their guarding abilities.

9. Gentle Nature: Despite their imposing look, they are generally described as gentle giants when well-socialized and properly taught. They can be good family pets if nurtured in a loving and nurturing setting.

10. Exercise and Care: Neapolitan Mastiffs require regular exercise to maintain them in good physical form, and they benefit from mental stimulation to prevent boredom. They also need special attention to the cleansing and upkeep of their skin folds to prevent skin disorders.

11. Health Concerns: Like many huge breeds, Neapolitan Mastiffs are prone to various health difficulties, including hip dysplasia, bloat, and skin problems due to their wrinkles. Responsible breeding and frequent veterinarian treatment are necessary to solve these challenges.

12. Short Lifespan: Unfortunately, Neapolitan Mastiffs have a somewhat short lifespan, often lasting approximately 7 to 9 years.

It's crucial to note that Neapolitan Mastiffs require early socialization and persistent, positive training to guarantee they become well-behaved and balanced dogs. They are a unique breed with special demands and features, and they may not be ideal for many households due to their size and guarding tendencies.

Temperament and Personality

The character and demeanor of a Neapolitan Mastiff can be highly different and unusual. These dogs have a combination of features that make them both protective and gentle when properly raised and socialized. Here are some major elements of their temperament and personality:

1. Protective: Neapolitan Mastiffs are naturally protective dogs. They have a strong instinct to preserve their family and territory. They are recognized for their courage and resolve when it comes to safeguarding their loved ones. This protective nature makes them great guard dogs and discourage prospective attackers.

2. Loyal: Neapolitan Mastiffs are highly loyal to their owners and families. They build profound ties with their human friends and are dedicated to them. They frequently display a strong feeling of loyalty and will do what it takes to protect and care for their family members.

3. Reserved with Strangers: While they are loyal and affectionate with their families, Neapolitan Mastiffs are often reserved and sometimes aloof with strangers. This reserved demeanor might make them ideal watchdogs, as they are inherently suspicious of individuals they do not know.

4. kind and Affectionate: Contrary to their intimidating appearance, Neapolitan Mastiffs may be kind and affectionate with their family members, particularly youngsters. They often prefer being close to their loved ones and may be quite affectionate when properly nurtured and socialized.

5. Calm Demeanor: Neapolitan Mastiffs are not energetic canines. They tend to have a quiet and laid-back personality, which can make them perfect for households searching for a dog that is not extremely energetic.

6. Stubbornness: Neapolitan Mastiffs can be rather stubborn, which makes regular and careful training vital. Positive reinforcement strategies and early socialization are vital to guarantee they become well-behaved and obedient pets.

7. Independence: They have a degree of independence in their character, which can make them less eager to please than certain other breeds. This means that they may not always respond instantly to commands, and they might be relatively self-reliant.

8. Needs Socialization: Proper socialization from an early age is crucial for Neapolitan Mastiffs. This helps them learn to be comfortable among different individuals and in varied situations, lowering their innate skepticism and guarding instincts when it's not essential.

9. Sensitivity: These dogs might be sensitive to their owners' emotions and moods, and they may respond to changes in the household environment. It's crucial to provide children with a secure and loving home.

In summary, Neapolitan Mastiffs are recognized for their protective and loyal attitude, which makes them wonderful guardians and dedicated family dogs. They have a calm disposition and may be friendly, but they also require early socialization, constant training, and awareness of their special needs to guarantee they become well-adjusted and well-behaved companions.

CHAPTER TWO
Education and Interaction

Training and socialization are key components of raising a Neapolitan Mastiff to ensure that they become well-behaved, balanced, and safe companions. Due to their protective and often stubborn temperament, it's necessary to start these processes early and apply positive reinforcement approaches. Here are some tips for teaching and socializing a Neapolitan Mastiff:

Training:

1. Start Early: Begin training your Neapolitan Mastiff as early as possible. Puppies are like sponges, and they can learn simple directions and habits fast. Early training helps develop a strong foundation.

2. Positive Reinforcement: Use positive reinforcement strategies, such as praise, treats, and awards, to encourage good conduct. Avoid strong penalties or physical corrections, as they might be counterproductive with this breed.

3. Consistency: Be consistent in your orders and expectations. Use the same cues and regulations, so your Mastiff understands what is expected of them.

4. Obedience Training: Enroll your Neapolitan Mastiff in an obedience training class. Professional trainers can help you work on commands like sit, stay, come, and leash walking. Consistent training will help your dog become well-mannered and responsive.

5. Socialize: Socialization is not just about introducing your Mastiff to different people and dogs; it's also about teaching them how to act appropriately in various settings. Take them to other areas, introduce them to new people and animals, and expose them to various sights and noises.

Socialization:

1. Early and Ongoing: Start socialization early, ideally during the puppy period, and continue throughout their lives. This is vital to help them become well-adjusted and less wary of strangers.

2. Exposure to Various Situations: Expose your Mastiff to a wide range of experiences, including automobile journeys, new surroundings, different sorts of people, and other animals. This helps children feel confident and comfortable in many circumstances.

3. favorable Interactions: Ensure that your Mastiff's early experiences with people and other dogs are favorable. This will assist diminish their natural wariness and make them more tolerant of new acquaintances.

4. Behavior Monitoring: Pay attention to your Mastiff's behavior during socializing. If they seem apprehensive or afraid, go at their pace and don't force interactions. Provide positive reinforcement for calm and confident demeanor.

5. Structured Play: Encourage your Mastiff to engage with other dogs in a controlled and supervised manner. This can help strengthen their social skills and lessen hostility or overprotectiveness.

6. Behavior Desensitization: Gradually introduce your dog to circumstances or objects that they might find threatening, like unfamiliar locations, loud noises, or weird objects. Reward calm and confident behavior during these experiences.

Remember that Neapolitan Mastiffs have a protective instinct, therefore it's vital to strike a balance between their protective nature and the requirement for socialization. Training and socialization should be continuous to ensure they grow into well-behaved and confident canines. If you're confused about how to teach and socialize your Mastiff, try talking with a professional dog trainer who has expertise working with huge, defensive dogs.

Exercise and Care

Proper exercise and care are necessary for preserving the health and well-being of a Neapolitan Mastiff. These dogs are enormous and powerful, and their distinctive features require specific attention. Here are some crucial factors for their exercise and care:

Exercise:

1. **Moderate Exercise:** Neapolitan Mastiffs are not overly active dogs, and they have a relatively modest energy level. However, they still require daily exercise to keep them in decent physical form. A daily stroll and some playtime in a properly fenced yard are generally plenty.

2. **Avoid Overexertion:** These dogs should not engage in intense exercise, especially during hot weather. Their loose skin might make them prone to overheating, so it's crucial to exercise them in the cooler hours of the day.

3. **Cerebral Stimulation:** In addition to physical activity, provide cerebral stimulation to prevent boredom. Puzzle toys, interactive activities, and training sessions can help keep young minds occupied.

Care:

1. **Grooming:** Neapolitan Mastiffs have loose, wrinkled skin that requires frequent maintenance. Clean and dry the skin folds to prevent skin infections or irritations. Regular brushing is also required to keep their short coat in good shape.

2. **Nutrition:** Feed your Neapolitan Mastiff a high-quality dog food appropriate for their age, size, and activity level. Be cautious of their weight to prevent obesity, which can lead to health difficulties.

3. **Health visits:** Schedule frequent veterinary visits to monitor your dog's health and handle any potential issues promptly. Neapolitan Mastiffs are prone to certain health difficulties such hip dysplasia and bloat.

4. **Dental Care:** Dental hygiene is crucial for all canines. Brush your Mastiff's teeth regularly and

provide dental chews or toys to help keep their teeth clean.

5. **Secure Enclosure:** Ensure that your yard is properly enclosed, as Neapolitan Mastiffs are robust and can be protective. This will prevent them from wandering and keep them safe.

6. **Training and Socialization:** As indicated previously, training and socialization are key components of care. Training helps create excellent behavior, while socialization ensures your dog is comfortable in diverse situations.

7. **Emotional Needs**: Neapolitan Mastiffs are loyal and thrive on human interaction. Spend quality time with your dog, and don't leave them alone for extended periods.

8. **Temperature Control:** These dogs are susceptible to excessive temperatures. In hot temperatures, give shade and access to fresh water. In cold weather, make sure they are shielded from the cold, as their short coat offers inadequate insulation.

9. **Pattern:** Establish a daily pattern for feeding, exercise, and other activities. Dogs, like Neapolitan

Mastiffs, thrive with predictability and constancy.

10. **Love and Attention**: Finally, remember that these dogs seek affection and attention. Provide love and constructive interactions to ensure their emotional well-being.

Neapolitan Mastiffs are known for their protective and devoted character, so taking excellent care of them and satisfying their individual needs is vital to maintaining a happy and healthy relationship with your dog.

CHAPTER THREE
Health and Common Concerns

Neapolitan Mastiffs are typically a healthy breed, although like any dogs, they are prone to some health disorders. It's crucial to be aware of these potential risks and to take precautionary steps. Some common health concerns in Neapolitan Mastiffs include:

1. **Hip Dysplasia:** This is a hereditary condition in which the hip joint doesn't grow properly. It can develop to arthritis and lameness. Responsible breeding techniques can help lower the risk of hip dysplasia.

2. Bloat (Gastric Torsion):
Neapolitan Mastiffs, like many large and deep-chested breeds, are prone to bloat. Bloat is a life-threatening condition in which the stomach fills with gas and twists on itself. It demands immediate veterinarian intervention.

3. Skin Issues: Neapolitan Mastiffs' loose, wrinkled skin can be prone to skin infections, particularly in the skin folds. Regular washing and upkeep of their skin are required to prevent skin issues.

4. Eye Issues: These dogs can be prone to different eye diseases, including entropion (a condition where the eyelids slide inward) and cherry eye (a prolapse of the third eyelid gland).

5. Heart Problems: Dilated cardiomyopathy, a disorder that affects the heart's ability to pump blood, can occur in Neapolitan Mastiffs. Regular cardiac examinations are advisable for this breed.

6. Elbow Dysplasia: Similar to hip dysplasia, elbow dysplasia is a hereditary disorder that affects the elbow joint. It can develop to lameness and arthritis.

7. Cancer: Neapolitan Mastiffs may be more prone to some types of cancer, such as mast cell tumors. Regular veterinary check-ups can help spot cancer early.

8. Hypothyroidism: This condition happens when the thyroid gland doesn't generate enough thyroid hormones. It can lead to different health complications and is typically addressed with medicine.

9. Obesity: Due to their low activity level, Neapolitan Mastiffs might be prone to obesity if their diet is not strictly maintained. Maintaining a healthy weight is vital for their overall well-being.

10.Breathing   Difficulties:
Neapolitan Mastiffs have a short muzzle, which can lead to breathing difficulties, particularly in hot or humid weather. It's crucial to keep them cool and well-hydrated in such settings.

To preserve your Neapolitan Mastiff's health:

• Choose a reputable breeder who does health exams on their breeding dogs to limit the possibility of genetic problems.

• Schedule regular veterinary check-ups and follow

recommended immunization and preventive care schedules.

• Provide a balanced diet and check their weight to prevent obesity.

• Pay attention to any signs of discomfort, suffering, or changes in behavior, and seek early veterinary care if you observe anything unexpected.

As with any dog breed, responsible breeding techniques, adequate nutrition, regular exercise, and careful care may go a long way in ensuring the health and lifespan of your Neapolitan Mastiff. Regular communication with your veterinarian is vital to address any particular health concerns or queries you may have regarding your individual dog.

The Neapolitan Mastiff as a Family Dog

Neapolitan Mastiffs can be great family dogs when properly nurtured, socialized, and trained. However, there are several factors and potential obstacles to keep in mind when choosing a Neapolitan Mastiff as a family pet:

Positive Aspects:

1. Loyal and Protective: Neapolitan Mastiffs are highly loyal to their families. Their inherent protective instinct can create an added sense of security for your household.

2. Kind and Affectionate: Despite their imposing appearance, Neapolitan Mastiffs may be kind and affectionate with family members, particularly children. They often create deep ties with their human counterparts.

3. Steady Temperament: These dogs often have a peaceful disposition, which can be a desirable feature in a family context. They are less likely to be highly energetic or hyperactive.

4. Good with Children: Neapolitan Mastiffs, when properly socialized, may get along well with children. They are usually patient and tolerant, making them a wonderful choice for families with kids.

5. Watchful and Deterrent: Their protective attitude can make them good watchdogs. Their very presence and menacing look can dissuade potential intruders.

Challenges to Consider:

1. Size and Strength: Neapolitan Mastiffs are enormous and powerful canines. It's crucial to ensure that they are well-trained and can be controlled, especially in situations where their size and power could be a worry.

2. Protectiveness: While their protectiveness is a benefit, it can also lead to overprotectiveness or violence if not properly managed. Socialization and training are necessary to ensure they don't become overly defensive.

3. Health and Lifespan: Neapolitan Mastiffs have a somewhat short lifespan, averaging about 7 to 9 years. This is something to consider if you're seeking for a long-term family companion.

4. Maintenance: Their unusual appearance with loose, wrinkled skin demands regular washing and maintenance to prevent skin concerns. Be prepared for grooming and skin fold care.

5. Exercise Needs: Neapolitan Mastiffs are not very active dogs, but they still need regular exercise to preserve their health. A daily stroll and playtime are often plenty.

6. Space: They demand space to move around comfortably, so living in a small apartment might not be suitable.

7. Socialization and Training: Neapolitan Mastiffs need early socialization and persistent, positive training to ensure they are well-behaved and well-adjusted in a household context.

In conclusion, a Neapolitan Mastiff may be a wonderful family dog provided you are committed to providing the essential training, socialization, care, and attention they require. They are protective, loyal, and cuddly, but their size and protective temperament must be regulated to provide a peaceful and safe family atmosphere. If you are contemplating this breed, it's crucial to research thoroughly, speak with breed specialists, and be prepared for the responsibilities that come with having a Neapolitan Mastiff.

The Neapolitan Mastiff in Modern Times

The Neapolitan Mastiff, also known as the Mastino Napolitano, has changed throughout the years and adapted to current circumstances, while preserving its particular qualities and historical value. Here are some traits of the Neapolitan Mastiff in current times:

1. Guardian & Protector: In modern times, Neapolitan Mastiffs continue to excel as guardians and protectors. Their imposing appearance, devotion, and protective instincts make them important assets for families and properties, particularly as watchdogs and deterrents against invaders.

2. Family pets: Many Neapolitan Mastiffs have converted from working dogs to loving family pets. When properly socialized and taught, they may be gentle and affectionate, making them excellent for families and children.

3. Therapy and Service Dogs: Some Neapolitan Mastiffs have found careers as therapy and service dogs. Their calm and steady demeanor can be beneficial in therapeutic settings, bringing comfort and support to individuals in need.

4. Conformation and Show Dogs: The breed is still actively shown in conformation dog shows. Breed lovers and breeders struggle to maintain the breed's standards and retain its unique appearance.

5. Rescue and Advocacy: In current times, there are rescue organizations and activists dedicated to the welfare and responsible breeding of Neapolitan

Mastiffs. These groups serve a critical role in preserving the health and well-being of the breed.

6. Health and hereditary Concerns: There is a growing awareness of the potential health difficulties linked with Neapolitan Mastiffs, and responsible breeders are making attempts to limit the occurrence of hereditary diseases through health testing and careful breeding techniques.

7. Social Media and Community: The emergence of social media has allowed Neapolitan Mastiff aficionados to interact and exchange knowledge about the breed, helping to promote responsible ownership and better care.

8. Education and material: There is a lot of material accessible for existing and potential Neapolitan Mastiff owners to learn about the breed's history, care, training, and health.

9. Legal and Ownership Considerations: In some places, there may be breed-specific legislation or rules surrounding ownership of Neapolitan Mastiffs or other large, powerful breeds. It's crucial for future owners to be informed of any such legal restrictions in their location.

Overall, the Neapolitan Mastiff has adapted to modern times by fulfilling different functions, including guardian, family companion, therapy dog, and show dog. Responsible breeding and education on the breed's particular qualities and demands have become increasingly vital in guaranteeing their well-being and promoting responsible ownership. While their historical role as protectors remains essential, they have also found a place as loving companions in many households throughout the world.

Conclusion

The Neapolitan Mastiff is a striking and intimidating breed with a rich history stretching back to ancient times. These canines are noted for their unusual appearance, protective temperament, and commitment to their families. In modern times, they continue to function as protectors, family companions, therapy dogs, and show dogs.

However, owning a Neapolitan Mastiff comes with certain

obligations. Proper socialization and training are vital to guarantee they are well-behaved and well-adjusted pets. They require regular care and attention to maintain their health and well-being, including grooming and monitoring for potential health issues.

While Neapolitan Mastiffs can be affectionate and gentle family members, their big size and protective instincts need be managed and channeled carefully. Responsible ownership and breeding procedures are crucial to preserve the breed's identity and limit the danger of hereditary health issues.

In the current period, the Neapolitan Mastiff has found a place in numerous roles and continues to be respected for its unique features. Whether working as a guardian, a therapy dog, or a cherished family member, these dogs bring a sense of security and loyalty to the households fortunate enough to have them.

THE END